Judit Szoó

Timeless health

A summary of my personal experiences with "earthing",
patching, cold therapy, and training.

Judit Szoó

Timeless health

Hernád, Hungary, EU - 2021

ISBN 978-615-01-0706-6

Facebook official site:

https://www.facebook.com/SzooJuditKilofaloKlub

Blog: http://szoojuditkilofalo.blogspot.com/

Instagram:

https://www.instagram.com/szoojuditkilofaloklub/

Content

INTRODUCTION

Who would not have dreamed of the possibility of eternal life, eternal youth, especially eternal health? Those who enjoy life and enjoy their days on Earth must have already pondered this topic.

I'm no exception myself: apart from a few more depressing periods that can be said to be natural, ☺ I basically love my existence. To learn, to understand, to be productive, and to live the many pleasures of life.

Eternal life is attractive when it applies equally to all people, for who wants to live alone for millennia while losing all their loved ones? Yet this is not the most important idea for me, because I have no problem with the normal, 80-100 year cycle of human life. What excites me much more is how to spend these decades in the most perfect condition, to preserve our strength, physical and mental freshness until the last moment, to drag the aging of our body and soul to the extreme, to extend it, to slow it down as much as possible?

For me, the issue of weight loss has always been related to this. I feel good when the image the mirror shows, is aesthetic according to my own values. I am fine when my life is harmonious. If I have peace of mind, I will not chew, I will not gnaw, I will not digest myself from within, if my principle of living is: do no harm to myself or my fellow human beings.

It tells a lot about me, that I stopped time when I was 38, and decided to stay that way from then on. ☺ At first, it was just for fun, later I became more and more convinced because I experienced, that age is just a number! And it's really important to my everyday well-being whether, say, at the age of forty, I talk about my former self as "when I was young" or "when I was a girl" (I always hear this in shock from women my age, because my grandmother used words like that!).

I feel totally different, my real life begins now: the children are adults, I am free again, but I am still really young enough to enjoy the world, to have my own programs independent of children.

I have definitely observed those who start to classify themselves as older around the age of forty, consistently calling twenty-thirty-year-olds "young" as if they themselves belonged to the same caste as retirees, both physically (in terms of fitness, appearance, state of health), and mentally starting to look more and more like the older age group!

I have been consciously fighting this since I was thirty-eight years old. ☺ I don't want to look or behave like a twenty year old! I don't deny the fact of aging, I don't even want to put my head in the sand. But I clearly feel, experience, it's up to me whether I feel young, perpetual, energetic, active, or weary, burnt out, "it hurts here - it hurts there" - an old woman: someone who has already given up life. I choose the former with complete determination, and it is no secret that I plan to "have" the same strength, fitness, muscle mass, performance, and last but not least, the aesthetic appearance already mentioned, even after many X.

So keeping the body young is one of my main topics, and nowadays as I see it, no matter what I want, for some reason my current life is about getting the most out of the issue, and gaining as much experience as possible.

The harmony of body and soul cannot exist without each other. In my previous volume, Fake hunger, I wrote about my experiences with emotional eating, and now I return to the integrity of the body: so let's see what I got!

"I am not a product of my
circumstances. I am a
product of my decisions."
(Stephen Covey)

BODY

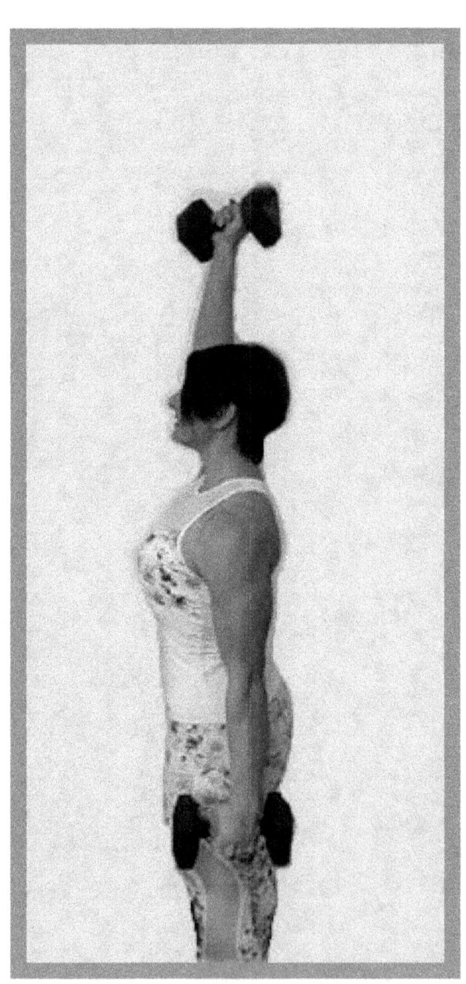

HISTORY

As I have already tangentially written about in my book Fake hunger, in the spring of 2020 I became more deeply acquainted with the work of Mr. Péter Lakatos. Péter is a coach, not a dietitian or doctor, as he often emphasizes, but reading his writings gives the impression and knowledge of a very wise person!

Why did I become interested in Peter's challenges? Because every novelty immediately excites me if it brings the promise of a healthy life, a healthy body, a youthful appearance and a hardened body.

As soon as we reach a level, we "settle" on it, it becomes a normal part of our lives, the challenge and the charm of novelty immediately disappears: we feel the urge to move to the next level, to cut into something new again! In January 2020, Péter Lakatos's "Intermittent Fasting or IF" became my new one.

First of all, I suggest that you read the content of https://timer12.hu/, then register! The program will be completely free, you will receive the tasks in e-mails for 12 weeks, starting from the basics, building on the steps of a higher level of lifestyle change. I also did this program back then and incorporated exciting new habits into my life.

(Note: it is possible that due to an update - development, the timer12.hu page will no longer be available in that form when my book is published. For more information, it is worth following Péter Lakatos's Facebook page!)

After 12 weeks, I looked more boldly at new challenges - also following Peter's writings - so I started with a combined cold therapy with "earthing", cold air therapy, and facial and body treatments with healing light, which I will write about in detail below.

All of the following tasks in order to:

- expand my boundaries
- do even more to maintain my health
- do everything I can to push out the visible and perceptible signs of aging
- to cheer up my days
- I feel like yes, I can even do that!

The year 2020, for one reason or another, will remain memorable for all of us. It has brought me all positive changes, on a self-knowledge, health and physical level.

Forced confinement provided a way to delve into my already popular topics, to realize my newer and newer ideas. I have never felt before so balanced and liberated. So let's see what led from April 2020, to this present state of Eden! ☺

„Take life in your own
hands, and what happens?
A terrible thing: no one
to blame."

(Erica Jong)

INTERMITTENT FASTING

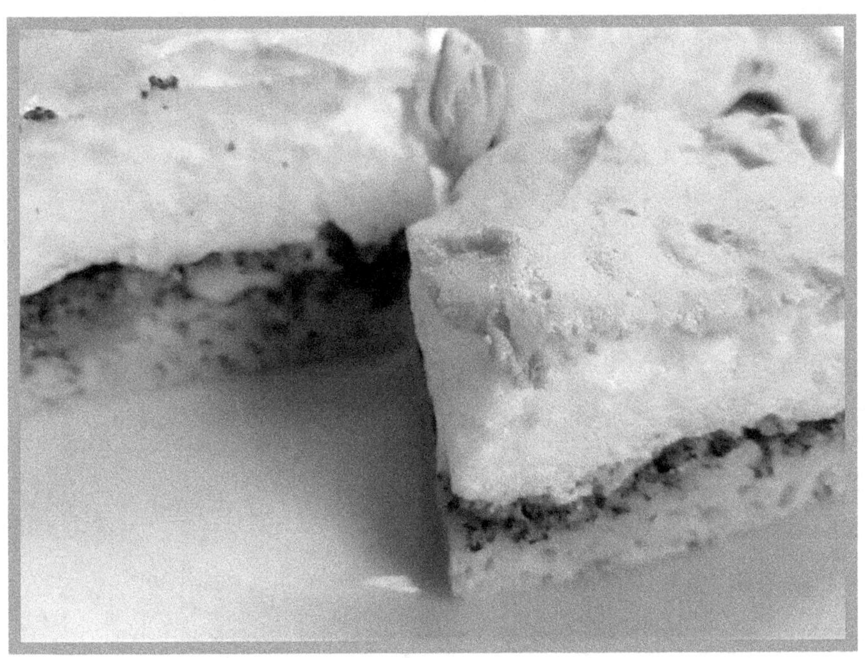

Based on the 12-week program of timer12.hu, I first introduced Intermittent Fasting (IF). The bottom line is to condense our meals into a specific time period of the day. If we opt for an 8-hour "time window," it means that our daily meals are limited to an 8-hour period of our choice. A lot of people have their first meal at noon, and the last one at 8 p.m.

But you can also choose to eat for the first time at 8 a.m. in the morning, and finish at 4 p.m. that day. It can be even stricter when you narrow the window to only 6 hours, in which case, for example, if you eat for the first time at 10 a.m. in the morning, you have to finish at 4 p.m. The 8-hour window is already considered advanced, for starters it is enough to eat in a 10-12 hour period.

What should you eat? If you have a proven diet, eat what is recommended in it. If you don't, just consume what you have eaten until then, acceptable if it's not "healthy", setting a time limit is sufficient at the beginning.

What is the point and advantage of this? You can find a lot of information about this in detail at Péter's site, but in essence, with the help of this method, you implement a periodic fast every day, as you load your body with food for 6-8 hours, then it gets 16-18 hours each time to rest, digest, and renew! Plus quite logically, in 8 hours you certainly can't (won't) eat as much food as you did before, possibly in 12-16 hours a day. This small change alone can result in weight loss.

„One always has to know when
a stage comes to an end. If
we insist on staying longer
then the necessary time, we
lose the happiness and the
meaning of the other stages
we have to go through."
(Paulo Coelho)

LIGHT, PATCHING, BREATHING

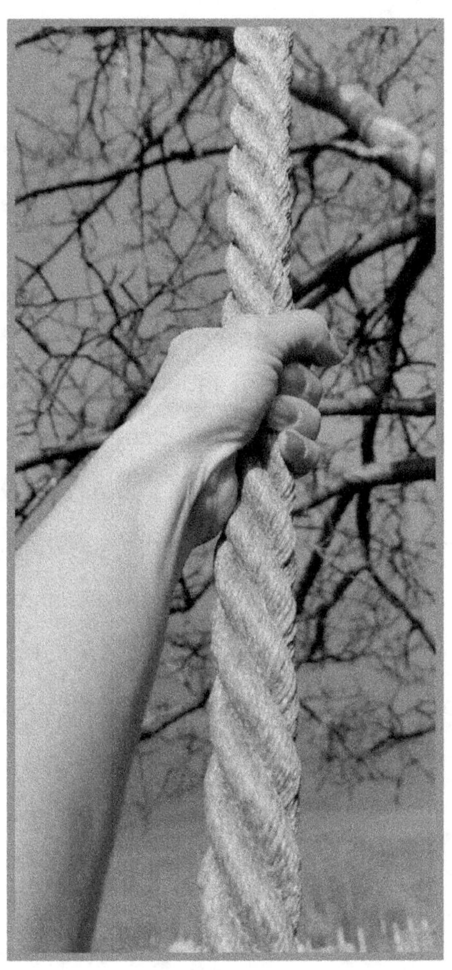

I have no intention to spoil all the surprises on timer12.hu's 12-week challenge, so all I mention is that, beyond the introduction of the time window:

- I also started to make sure I didn't lie down with a full stomach.

- In the evening, I dimmed the lights in our home to prepare the body for the rest period. For this I downloaded a free software to my computer: https://iristech.co/iris-mini/?fbclid=IwAR3Z1pNVEL0QA7Vij_DRInyB1QzEnDfN ne71qBtntUeMWG_TI89JwDqVmzk And more modern phones and tablets already have a "built-in" blue light filter function.

- I introduced sunbathing. Yes, even in the cold. For beginners, you "show" yourself to the Sun for 10-15 minutes a day (even if you don't see it, so even in cloudy weather...). With as large a free surface area as possible: I didn't overdo it, in case of better weather, I rolled up the sleeve of my sweater, but I thought continuity was the point, and to start the whole process at all.

- I closed my evening showers with a 30 second jet of cold water. I couldn't turn the tap completely cold, even in "half-cold" position it was a horrible experience to be honest, but I kept doing it persistently because I believed in its effect. I will write about these in more detail.

- I slept with a patch on my mouth at night. This is where Buteyko breathing comes into play, which is the basis of everything. As long as breathing isn't okay, it's almost unnecessary to start anything, but of course - it's not that extreme. Simply put, proper breathing is considered nasal breathing. In English, if you pay attention (especially if you've been mouth-breathing so far) and consciously concentrate on taking and exhaling air only on your nose, at a more controlled, slower pace, you've already done a lot for your health! Night patching, among other things, plays a major role in eliminating / reducing snoring, dry mouth and nasal congestion. Buteyko course can also be taken, you will find all the necessary information about it on the net.

- As well as why it is recommended to learn how to breathe properly. And for patching, we use a skin-friendly adhesive patch: look for it as a "3M Micropore" patch, completely anti-allergenic, cheap, each roll lasts long enough. Some practical tips for using the patch correctly:

- A torn strip can be used several times in a row. In the morning you glue it to the edge on a non-textile surface (e.g. alarm clock, bedside lamp base, edge of a bedside table), in the evening you simply pull it off from there, and use it.

- When you tear off a piece, fold and glue both ends of the strip back under the two edges, on a few millimeters of surface: this is so that in the morning, when you want to take it off, you don't have to "scrape" it off your face at the edges. The small, non-sticky handles will help to avoid this problem.

- In the same way, always fold back the end of the tape on the roll: the next time you tear, you don't have to search for minutes where the end is stuck.

- When you tear a new strip, stick it on your palms or arms, and pull it off right away (as if it were a light waxing) this way it will lose a little of its strong adhesive power. This will help to preserve the skin on your lips, and prevents dryness as well.

- If it does, the lipstick is the perfect solution, even when applied just before patching. By following these, you won't even notice that you're sleeping with a patch: the experience of many of us, is that in the morning, we only realize that it's on us, when we want to speak, and we don't succeed. ☺

- Last but not least, at timer12.hu another task was to be barefoot outdoors, to come into contact with the Mother Nature with bare feet, if only for a few minutes. In the first round I could not try this lesson (since it was winter when the challenge started...)

"Man is the measure of all
things, of things that are
that they are, and of things
that are not that they are
not."

(Protagorasz)

E A R T H I N G

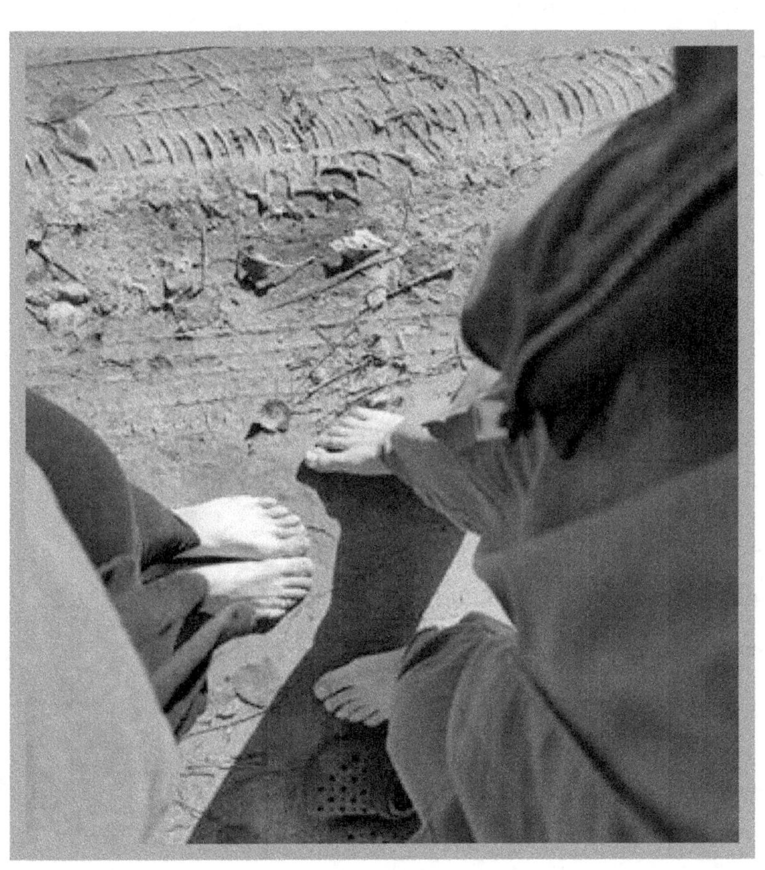

But winter doesn't last forever either, so when it comes to "earthing", my time has come! On March 19, my birthday, I was past several occasions.

First, let's see - what is grounding? In ordinary language, it means that your bare skin and soles are in contact with the ground (the motherland) while walking. More scientifically, e.g. according to the information on *hegylakomagazin.hu*, "the technique called "earthing "has an anti-inflammatory, muscle-strengthening effect and also reduces oxidative stress in the cells."

According to some research, if our skin comes in contact with the ground, it has a health-enhancing effect because the Earth, as a planet, has its own electron charge. "*These free electrons from the soil, when they get through the skin into the body, function as a natural antioxidant, thereby reducing inflammation and balancing cortisol levels, thus reducing stress and improving the quality of our sleep.*"

Furthermore, the electrons released from the earth can also be effective against joint pain, and walking barefoot changes the electrical activity of the brain: we become more alert and energetic. It also increases blood circulation, so it has a beneficial effect on the cardiovascular system.

And why I especially like the fact that the unevenness of the soil, stones, pebbles, smaller twigs massage all the muscles of the sole, the point of acupressure, thus increasing the function, blood circulation and immunity of the internal organs.

This was the "official" definition, but let's see how was I personally experiencing grounding?

So I started in the spring, when the air was so warm at times that we could go to our favorite forest in a t-shirt, accompanied by our two German Shepherd dogs. I remember the first time I slipped out of my slippers, I felt like a world-saving hero who was just writing history and taking on the dangerous unknown, taking on the role of a weirdo in the eyes of "normal" people as well. ☺ After all, it's really not an ordinary thing in our civilized world to walk barefoot in public, in an environment where it's not common (no one on a beach would feel like a world-saving hero because that's where it's accepted).

It was a very pleasant feeling. My feet never hurt, nor any other part of my heels or feet, maybe my "athletic" past or rather my present, also played a role in this. It was especially nice to walk and get up on the sometimes cool and sometimes lukewarm forest ground. In shady parts, the soil was compact, solid, with its own natural unevenness, which I enjoyed separately, thinking about how thoroughly the reflex points of my foot are massaged at that time. And in a sunny area, the sandy soil was dry and lukewarm, reminiscent of the beach, and in some cases I sank to my ankles, which had a positive effect on the sense of balance.

Around us is the awakening spring nature, budding, fresh green foliage trees, birds chirping of indescribable beauty, butterflies... Not to mention the emergence of deer, fat forest rabbits, the distinctive sound of pheasants that always brought our dogs euphoric excitement. The medium itself is so relaxing, but when you come in contact with the bare ground, you almost blend in with nature.

In addition, my husband and I take part in our world-saving thoughts, our visions for the future. We give thanks for the present, first for each other, for our values (health, happiness, harmonious life, beautiful home, successful children, good human relationships, work we are happy to do, thanks for the food, opportunities, garden, forest, animals, casual schedule), which we can live in. And for our youth, our physique, and that we could start a whole new life with each other, and finally, that we could learn from all the mistakes of our previous marriages.

Even if we start out a little cold or depressed, it is absolutely certain that we will come home fully charged, exchanged, excited - and since we already know exactly how this works, it can't happen that we simply "don't feel like" starting, because we already know that the end matters, and that is guaranteed to be good. ☺

I didn't feel any particular change from the barefoot walk itself. I did it because it was good, and especially because I believed I was doing myself good with it: I believe that anything that leads back to a natural lifestyle, can only benefit me! Natural foot massage alone can only have a positive effect, especially if I even add reflex zone points!

Just as our feet are a mini "map" of our entire body, so is the palm, face, or cochlea, for me these are all fantastically exciting ways to maintain and improve the health of my body.

Well, on second thought, there is a definite change though: in the morning, until I have started "earthing", both of my legs, the outer edge of my soles, and sometimes the soles themselves, often hurt. Then it became ok, after a few minutes, but until then, the first few steps were unpleasant. Since almost a year of "earthing", this complaint has completely disappeared, my feet never hurt again.

As the weather warmed up, and the summer months were approaching fast, we walked more and more on barefoot. I was soon joined by my husband, who was happy to follow me in trying out the new trends I had discovered.

<u>"Earthing" videos on YouTube:</u>

Walking bare feet in January | Ep. 1

https://www.youtube.com/watch?v=KhIwh9IvIm8&t=232s&ab_channel=Sz o%C3%B3JuditKil%C3%B3fal%C3%B3

How much can I eat for lunch, what cookies I like, and how to ask the Universe? | Ep. 2

https://www.youtube.com/watch?v=1QlFxx0IOAg&t=19s&ab_channel=Szo %C3%B3JuditKil%C3%B3fal%C3%B3

C O L D   T H E R A P Y

- **Cold "earthing"**
- **Cold alternating shower**
- **Cold air bath**

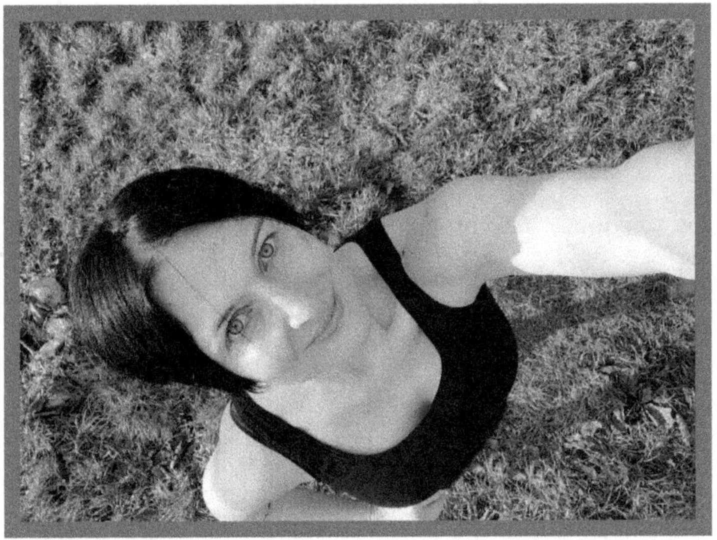

The photo was taken on December 9, after 20 minutes outside…

With the onset of autumn, an exciting change began. The cool weather has arrived! I tried to find information on how to get one's body used to cold "earthing" without suffering injuries, but unfortunately I did not find the kind of "mouth-watering", detailed, step-by-step "literature" I would have needed on the subject.

Because I love discovering new things, I had no difficulty at all, in taking on the role of the "experimental rabbit" again, and embarking on the new challenge of experiencing this journey myself! ☺

First of all, considering the practical part of earthing, the easiest way is to choose a comfortable garden rubber slipper as footwear. There may be sections where - e.g. because of the passing of a car - on a narrow forest road you have to step aside from the sandy ground to the gravelly, rougher part of the road with the dogs: then it is easiest to step back in the slippers to avoid injuries rather than constantly putting on shoes. The slippers can be carried in one hand while walking anyway, but in the case of a backpack of the right size, we can also put it in it, or we can throw a ribbon on our shoulders, whichever is more suitable for the body.

I started cold grounding around September-October, proceeding with natural and gradual cooling. Since I've been walking barefoot in the woods (since spring) my feet (and my whole body as well) had a way of getting used to the increasingly cool conditions. In the early autumn, the barefoot walk didn't mean any breakage, the ground was cooler, no doubt, I had to get used to the fact that there was no dusty sand on any section of the road, except for that, I could still stay within my comfort zone.

On the first really cold day, I experienced the following: for the first time, I only felt cold flowing from the ground through my feet. As I progressed the distance I traveled, a pleasant tingling-numbing feeling ran through my feet, which then passed into something as if I were constantly stepping on tiny, pungent crumbs of gravel, such as when we were walking on an asphalt road, for example. Of course, there was no crush on the dirt road: the cold, the agitation of the blood circulation, I suppose, was accompanied by such a feeling.

After about 1.5 km (0.9 mile) we reached an overpass, where - precisely because of the certain asphalt-gravel road - we had to take the slippers back for a few minutes.

This time was just enough for our feet to rest, warm up a bit, and then, after the overpass we could continue the barefoot walk. Usually from then on, I could only feel the pleasant tingling, and although the ground never "warmed up" under my feet, it was still nice to make my way barefoot despite the cool.

I must mention here, it was another milestone from spiritual point of view: just as in the summer, contrary to generally accepted social customs, I began to walk barefoot, despite many people gave me the weird look. Some even asked: "Isn't it enough to be without shoes, you even want to catch cold?!" or "Shall I buy you a pair of shoes?" Because of course, when we met other hikers who came dressed to the top, in scarves, boots, big coats, looked at us like the "weird couple" with widened eyes, and there were those who even asked ironic questions. In this case, of course, we did not start a long lecture, rather gave short answers about the excellent immune-boosting, circulatory-improving effect, and the significantly increase in the ability to tolerate stress. But inside, I must admit, I just felt like a world-conquering empress again. ☺ ☺ ☺

This transient temperature persisted for a few weeks, and each time I walked longer distances, with less and less feeling of cold or tingling - as did my husband.

And when the first real winter day dawned, when the puddles of the forest were covered with ice all the way, and the trees were covered in hoarfrost, well, there my world-conquering self, beat her chest a little quieter... But we set off (my husband didn't dare take on the mission at first, he stayed in his boots), but I wanted to try, that was the point, continuity, because my end goal was walking in the snow! And that requires fitness, so it was not worth missing out on steps. And in general, these things that force me out of the real comfort zone were the most exciting for me: to expand, to push the limits of my tolerance!

Here again, a little help would have come in handy, but I didn't even find the details of this at Péter's works, so after gaining some suitable icy experience, I made the following discoveries, which I can pass on to anyone who would like to try cold therapy grounding.

1. Dress in layers, you should not feel cold! It is more than enough for the first time that you are walking barefoot in winter! The goal is to strengthen your immune system, your stress tolerance, your health and fitness, not to die. ☺ I wore pants, a thin top, a T-shirt, a long-sleeved turtleneck on my upper body, two thin sweatshirts and a thicker warmer top. At first, I even wore gloves. ☺

2. Get out of your slippers and walk barefoot in the first round, until your feet start to hurt or burn uncomfortably! Pain is always a sign! It doesn't have to hurt, it shouldn't. The good tingling, similar sensation to touching little pebbles, or pleasant numbness are acceptable but if it hurts, maybe your fingers become numb, you need to rest: just step back in your slippers! The cold therapy part will be plentiful (wearing slippers without socks, in the middle of winter, in the woods!) ☺ you just pause the grounding part a bit.

3. For me 10 minutes was usually enough, you can feel exactly when the soles had enough rest, when life "come back into them," when they warm up so much that you can step on the cold ground again.

4. In very cold, a 10-minute grounding is usually followed by a 10-minute slipper walk. But there is no rule here, it entirely depends on your level of comfort: if you prefer the ratio of two minutes barefoot, 15 minutes of slippers walking, that's fine too. This is the normal part of "training", there is no good or bad here, we only pay attention to the feedback of the body because we do not want to cause injury or harm, but to build, improve, strengthen, develop.

5. The more winter barefoot walks you go, the better your body adapts to the cold. There will also come a day, when a single step back in the slippers will be enough for a full walk. And finally, you will be able to walk the entire distance with your bare feet without stopping.

6. How far should you walk? It again, depends on your level of comfort.

Preferably, as far as you can go. ☺ We are lucky enough to live next to the forest, so we could practically walk for days without stopping. The ideal distance for us has been 6 km (3.7 miles). The dogs also have a chance to run around, while we are slowly overwhelmed by the pleasant fatigue, but it is no less worthwhile for someone to be able to do 2-3 kilometers (1-2 miles).

7. What should be the pace? It again, depends on your level of comfort. This should be about you, not about expectations. We decided on a brisk walk. When we can still talk, but here and there we have to gasp for air. But if you admire the scenery, and prefer slow pace, there's nothing wrong with it either: the point is you do it!

8. How to breathe? Referring to Peter, nasal breathing is the absolute thing to follow. (Every time, in general.) That's what I strive for, even though, if I talk in the meantime, it's not easy at all. ☺ I don't do separate Buteyko exercises like I wrote, neither does my husband.

It doesn't take me long to consciously pay attention to nasal breathing and reducing its frequency. I use abdominal breathing (so your chest won't move up and down) and say 4 sec inhalation - 2 sec hold - 6 sec exhale. If you walk alone and in a less crowded part, you can even apply a patch. We also talk in the meantime, we also meet people, so this is not the way for us.

9. How often should you walk barefoot in winter? It again, depends on your level of comfort. In very cold weather, you won't want it every day, I can tell you. With us, the system has developed in such a way that from October to February, one walk a week (Sunday, when we both have a day off in training). By the time this day comes, we gradually get excited about it, because we know that the experience will recharge us in an incredible way. Then, of course if it is light weather or the sun is shining and it makes us feel good, we go several times a week. To make sense, I see a minimum of one occasion a week during the winter months.

10. What to do after you get home from a walk? First, wash the feet of course, I always do it with cold water (soap, nail brush). Why in cold water?

    Because the heat causes them to hurt and gives a burning feeling. Plus, you can further increase the desired good effects of cold therapy.

11. For the same reason, stay barefoot even after washing your feet. If you have a cold, paved, stony surface at home, feel free to walk on it without socks and slippers! You'll be surprised, that after an hour and a half of barefoot forest walks the once ice-cold stone will feel pleasantly lukewarm. ☺ The best option for continuing in-house cold therapy.

12. IMPORTANT NOTE! Everything I have described is based on my own experience! I am healthy, I can do all these without difficulty and negative consequences. But of course, everyone should be judge these based on their own limitations or possibilities! If you catch cold all the time - practice at your own risk! Always, in all circumstances, a sober mind should lead you and pay attention to the clear feedbacks of your body!

13. I also think as always, that only what we do with good feelings can have a positive effect on us! If you usually sit in three sweaters in your apartment with the heating up, it may not be your way at the moment.

You have to want it too, but voluntarily, it should be a bit hard to achieve, but enjoy it more than you hate it, look forward the next experience, and feel like a hero when you did it. As long as that is the case, you are on the right track. ☺

And after many month of dry, rarely rainy winter weather, the day finally dawned when so much snow fell at night that I could even try walking in the snow in a bikini, on January 25, at 0 C!

It happened in the morning, right after waking up. At first, it didn't cause any shock to walk in the snow, it was especially pleasant. The wind blew relatively hard that day, which intensified the feeling of cold. For the first time though, I was able to spend 12 minutes in the snow, barefoot, almost without clothes. ☺ I didn't suffer any harm , ☺ I didn't get sick, I didn't catch a cold, I have been feeling perfectly ever since. It felt really good to do, to try.

A video on these challenges has also been produced for YouTube:

https://www.youtube.com/watch?v=KhIwh9IvIm8&t=229s&ab_channel=Szo%C3%B3JuditKil%C3%B3fal%C3%B3

So far on the subject of cold earthing. I have described everything about my cold therapy practices (of which the cold alternating shower and the cold air bath will follow), I will summarize their (based on my experiences) beneficial effects in a separate chapter.

You can watch my first YouTube video of my snowy bikini experience here:
In a bikini in the snow! | Intact. 3
https://www.youtube.com/watch?v=je6m2rxttT4&t=2s&ab_channel=Szo%C3%B3JuditKil%C3%B3fal%C3%B3

Cold alternating shower

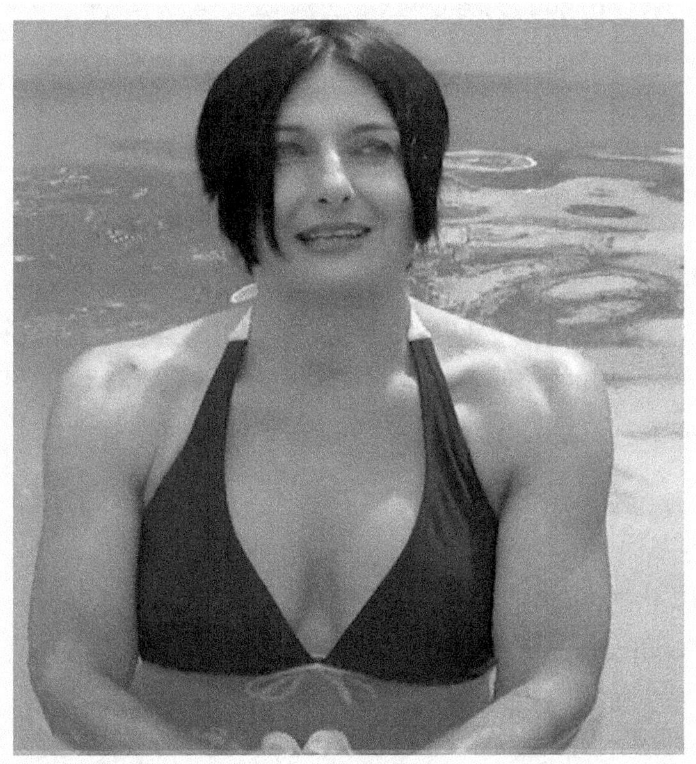

Together with the timer12.hu program, as I mentioned earlier, I introduced a 30-second cold shower to finish my baths with.

It was hell. ☺ I've tried to love it, but there's not much to love about the fact, that after the comfortable warm water, you turn the lever to pound ice-cold water on yourself. I'm not saying it doesn't feel good afterwards, but experiencing it isn't something pleasant.

As the months passed, as always, life showed the next step. From Ms. Kinga Perjés (a nutrition expert / lifestyle consultant), I read about the process of the three-round hot and cold shower. I tried it that day, and it proved so successful that I've only done it that way, ever since! With this method, you can get there without further ado to even enjoy the process!

In connection with the cold shower, Kinga and Péter Lakatos also refer to Dutch extreme athlete Wim Hof, who became famous for bathing in icy lakes and rivers, running marathons in the desert without drinking, but also mentions his famous breathing practice. He claims that anyone is capable of these achievements and has also developed his own method, which consists of special breathing techniques, cold bath exercises.

Thai chi and yoga. All this proves that human tolerance can be extended to extreme limits and we can influence the biochemical processes in our bodies with our minds. According to him, health is a normal state of human beings, and we are all able to use his methods to "self-heal".

I don't do it regularly, but I have tried a method of breathing that he claims to create positive stress for the body, making us more resistant to everyday stressful situations, increasing adrenaline levels, alleviating inflammation and pain. It helps regeneration in athletes, otherwise the sleep quality of those affected improves, it also has a positive effect on depression. Not only breathing alone, but the whole lifestyle helps with this.

We can't - and maybe don't even need it first - dive in icy lakes, but for starters, a hot and cold shower is perfect. The positive effects of this (and of regular cold therapy in general), in addition to what Wim Hof has said above, could be the following in general (My personal experiences will be described in a later chapter):

1. Increases blood circulation in athletes, so it delivers more oxygen to the muscles, which accelerates regeneration and increases performance.
2. It helps to eliminate cellulite: it tightens and smoothes the skin and rejuvenates it in general, the cells are almost renewed.
3. Increases energy consumption. Péter Lakatos writes about white and brown adipose tissue in several places. White stores energy, brown can burn it: it helps regulate energy use and body temperature. However, with increasing age, this adipose tissue decreases, which explains the obesity associated with aging. But a cold shower activates brown adipose tissue, so you already have a fantastic solution by introducing a cold shower on how to eliminate obesity over the years!
4. Strengthens the heart
5. Reduces the symptoms of diabetes
6. Strengthens the immune system
7. Antidepressant effect
8. Better sleep quality
9. The otherwise cold limbs become warm
10. Digestion will be better

11. Frontal sensitivity, tendency to migraine may decrease

12. Better metabolism

13. Better cold tolerance, decreasing heat demand, i.e. we can feel comfortable in the room at lower temperatures

So I do the cold shower process as follows. First, I open the bathroom window and turn off the heating. It is not a requirement, but it makes sense to me. I do the necessary bathing in normal temperature water. Then the actual therapy begins: I turn up the temperature of the water with the tap until it almost burns.

I shower all over my body from ankle to neck. When I reach the limit of my tolerance, I turn the lever in the cold direction, but only halfway, not yet completely to the stop. Why? Because in the first round, after the hot feeling, the cold water is so brutally cold (it seems) that it effectively hurts my knees, and my bones as I water my body, but if it is only half cold at first, it is not. Of course, if you don't experience this, you've can turn it to completely cold in the first round. ☺

I also start with cold water from my left ankle: I keep moving upwards, I don't have to soak an area for long. Legs, knees, thighs, abdomen. Bottom again, but now the back of the leg as well: heel, calf, back thigh, buttocks. It comes from the right leg in the same way, then left arm from wrist to shoulder, right arm, and finally chest-back. In principle, the chest should be the last, but I don't usually make a difference there. If I had it and it was good, I could still sprinkle myself back and forth with the cold water, then set it to lukewarm, normalize my condition a bit, and start rolling towards the warmer ones again. For the second time, I'm setting the temperature completely cold, and I'm moving up from my left ankle in the same way. Although it is much colder water than at first, it is still pleasant, because overheated skin is especially good for cooling. When I'm done with the themed cooling, I just run the cold on myself again, until it's good and start the last, finishing round. Which is always cold!

When you get out of the shower after that, it's like you're reborn. ☺ The good thing about this is (just like with cold earthing) that it doesn't distract you from the fact that not every moment is pleasant in the meantime, but you already know how fantastic it will be afterwards, so you do it again and again.

When should this be done? For me, the most ideal thing is to do it after a morning workout, because with the euphoria caused by the workout and the heat shock caused by the hot and cold water, I get enough energy to feel like I can fly. In the meantime, I read that it is not necessarily good and recommended to do it immediately after training to cool the warm muscles. However, in case of sports injuries, immediate ice baths, cooling and icing, are recommended for a regenerative purpose.

In the evening it is no different, which can be a problem because we should prepare the body to fall asleep. But we managed to find a solution by taking a shower relatively early in the evening, and go to bed hours later, by then our waking state will return to normal.

How many times should you do it? There is no rule for this.

I think the more times, the more effective that is, even every single day. But if you can only get yourself to it every two days or twice a week, you already do it twice as often as an average person who never does. ☺

By what method? It depends on your preferences. I prefer the three turns, but my husband only undertakes one turn: he sets the water temperature very warm, then turns it to completely cold, and he doesn't go through it methodically from wrist to shoulder, ankle to abdomen like I do. He immediately starts from the top of his head and just lets it go down everywhere. He prefers this method. In terms of the end result, his experience is similar to mine. So, your job is to find out how it works best for you, for example, there is nothing wrong with closing a normal shower with a 30 second cold water "rinse" because that is already a fantastic feeling!

Cold air bath

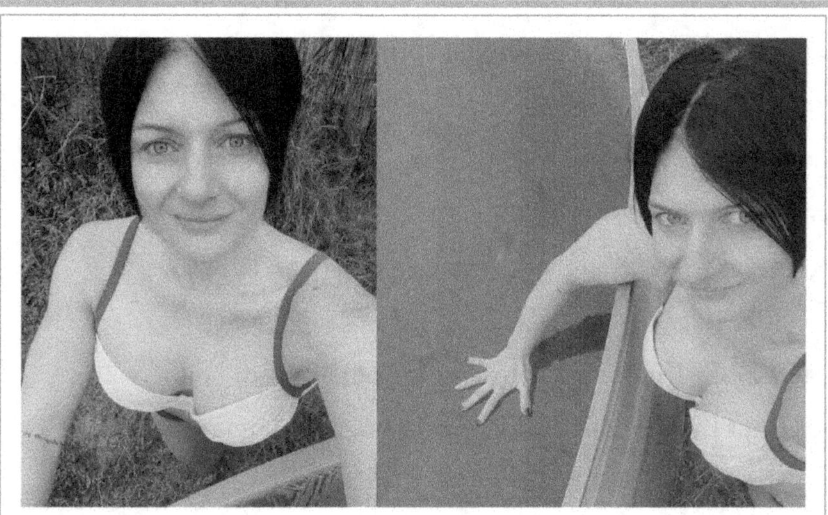

2020. december 27.
- 4 C fok

After cold earthing, and a hot-cold alternating shower, we have arrived at the third major strength test, cold air therapy (or cold air bath).

Before I read about the positive effects of *cold air therapy* in a post, I didn't think much about this topic. Based on this logic, the sauna is *hot air therapy*. But both are equally good for the body, to increase durability and the level of tolerance. So again, all I needed was one of Péter Lakatos' posts, in which I spotted the term "cold air therapy", and I knew right away that I was lost again! ☺ Here was the new challenge ☺

Unfortunately, Péter did not share the details on this either, I tried to put the process together from fragments, and based on this, the implementation developed for me as follows:

I soon realized that contact with cold air is most effective when we leave as much skin surface as possible uncovered. Nevertheless, to get used to it, 20 minutes was enough in our garden in a casual pants and a thin hoodie in the middle of winter. For the second time, I went out after waking up, all my clothing were a short nightgown and an open robe (barefoot, in garden slippers...) It was cold, but the sun was exceptionally sunny, I could even sunbathe my face a little.

On this occasion, after 20 minutes, I felt it was enough. This happened in early December at temperatures around +3 degrees Celsius. ☺

For the third time, I wore knee pants and a leotard during the day, without sunshine and in light winds. It was here that I first realized that the cold air bath provides an opportunity for a fantastic outdoor workout. Knowing these, this is how I can summarize how I think it is worth doing and building this.

1. First of all, a cold air bath can also be started in your home, especially if you do not live in a house with a garden... In the morning you can stand on the balcony. You can train with an open window! You can take a shower with the window open or with an open window, you can do really anything inside the apartment, increasing the duration of ventilation.

2. Then: air bathing is not the same as standing still and slowly freezing to death. ☺ In other words, no one forbids us to make any kind of movement! During the air bath for the first time, I just stood there, walking up and down in the garden, stroking the dogs. I got bored of these very soon, and only five minutes passed, and I felt terribly cold.

That's why I started to prune raspberry bushes, rake, sweep leaves, cut back flowers, collect dog feces, so get myself moving! Twenty minutes flew unnoticed! ☺ The next time I didn't feel like doing any of these, and obviously I ran out of these things after a while, so I realized: I'm going to train! Strange as it may seem, you only have to "survive" the cold for the first 5 minutes, after that it feels like a switch is turned on in you, and your internal heat source starts to work, the feeling of discomfort disappears and you move around as easily as if you were in a heated room! Since I train regularly, it wasn't hard to get some exercises out of my head: I squatted, I did breakouts, I climbed a rope. I warmed up to feel nothing of the cold of winter, and my childhood memories of "wintering" outside immediately jumped in, when we froze in the school yard at the beginning of class, and by the end of class we felt almost spring from a lot of movement...

3. What is the ideal duration? Obviously, the more you adapt, the longer you last, and the less you feel uncomfortable, stressful. The expert suggests to stay until you start shivering, which can be 3-4 minutes.

So if you go out in a leotard and endure a few minutes, you're already a hero. ☺ It can be raised continuously later! I don't think it's worth forcing, if it doesn't feel good. This is true for everything in the world! Well-being, long life, good health can be created in a thousand other ways, cold therapy is not necessarily everyone's ideal way there. ☺

4. How often should you do this? You would never guess: it depends on your level of comfort. In really cold winter, I think once a week is quite enough, especially if you do other cold therapy things as well. Of course, you would like it more often, fell free to do it as many times as you want! Go on polar bears! ☺

"Judith, aren't you afraid of catching cold?" I was asked several times as I told people about my experiences with the cold. No, was not scared at all. I always pay attention to the reactions of my body. A pleasant tremor, minimal discomfort is part of the normal procedure: we expand the boundaries, strengthen the body's resilience, the immune system. On the other hand, when the cold is uncomfortable, "it hurts", I feel bad, or the cold shakes my body, etc...

I know that's enough, and then I stop. But frankly, I didn't worry too much about it. I wasn't afraid of catching a cold either, because I think if you gradually increase your time in the cold, your body has a way to get used to it. In addition, (I read this explanation in an article), that it is not the cold air that makes us sick when seasons change, (entering from winter to spring, summer from autumn), but the weakened immune system cannot cope with viruses, bacilli, bacteria in the air, and those make us ill. Of course, I can't stress enough to anyone to take into account their own tolerance and build, before start making friends with the cold, be it water or air. Strange as it may seem, since the cold is not a pleasant feeling at all, you should still enjoy it to some extent. ☺ You can't go without it. I can't even take cold air therapy at any time (go out in a bikini in winter) or take a hot-cold alternating shower! I don't know the reason yet, I think it can be related to fatigue and exhaustion, but I just skip that part for 2-3 days. Then it turns to the other extreme, I am constantly craving the "cold" in any form for up to a week. As long as we pay conscious attention to the messages of the body, I don't think there can be a problem.

Who is cold therapy not recommended for?

For patients with fever, heart disease and high blood pressure.

"Emotions are like waves.

You can't stop them,

but you decide which one to ride. "

(unknown)

Hot air bath

(sauna)

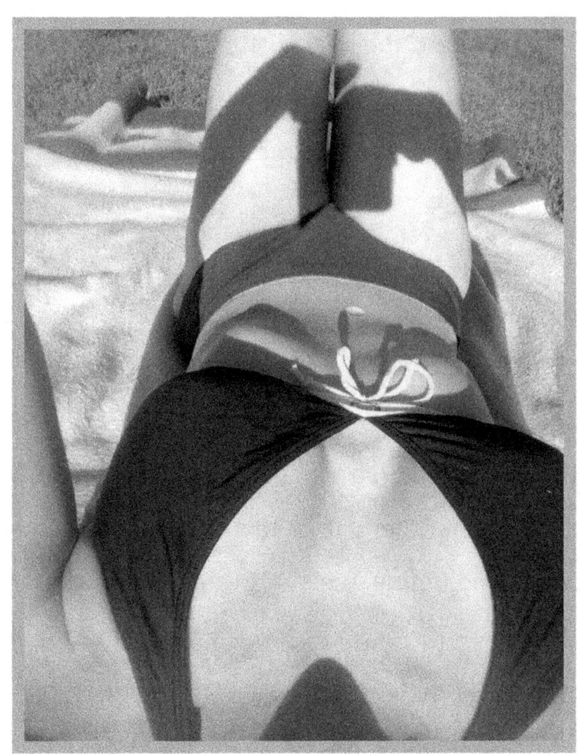

You may be wondering why I am writing about the hot sauna in the cold therapy section, but it will soon be clear why this is also related to the topic.

First of all, as I wrote earlier, this is also air therapy, just not cold but hot.

We know much more about the health effects of the sauna (based on decades of research) than about the cold:

1. Regular sauna users are less affected by heart problems in older age.
2. It lowers blood pressure.
3. It has a good effect on rheumatic diseases
4. The detoxifying effect has long been known (nothing complicated: with sweating during training)
5. High heat puts a strain on the body, so the time spent in the sauna is equivalent to a low-intensity cardio workout: in the meantime, the heart rate will be faster and stay that way for a while, even after using the sauna. This is also fantastic, because as a beginner, or someone having an injury, the effect of cardio training can be achieved by simply having a sauna.
6. Increases growth hormone levels associated with faster regeneration (e.g. in athletes)

I had a sauna experience with my husband for the first time. I didn't like it at all. ☺ When I was a kid, I couldn't take an inhalation either (when you lean over a bowl full of hot chamomile tea, and you put a big towel on your head as a cover. At the time, we used this to cure a cold, but I couldn't stand it for more than a second, because I was drowning in the hot steam).

The sauna wasn't a much better experience either: in addition to being terribly warm, the thirst for fresh air appeared as well. Luckily, we started with short periods of time, when the heat became unbearable, we came out immediately. After that, I did not even consider cold water immersion seriously, a quick, cold shower was maximum I could tolerate.

But it is all a matter of habit and practice. We went to the sauna regularly and we gradually increased the time spent there and then got used to the subsequent cooling.

When I first dived into the cold water pool, up to the level of my shoulder and I couldn't silently endure the ordeal. ☺ For the second time, I was just yelling inside, ☺ and from time to time I spent a few seconds more in the pool.

Eventually I got to a higher level and I could spend minutes immersing myself in the cold water: those moments were especially cold while I let myself dip in and out in the water, but being in the water - literally - breathlessly, I floated motionless in it, and suddenly there was complete calm and peace in me! *The previously painfully icy water became completely neutral, I felt like I could spend hours in it, without feeling unwell.*

The minutes and hours after the dive are euphoric! After a hot sauna-cold dive combination, you feel just like after a hot-cold alternating shower! It's as if you've done an exhausting exercise, and the well-deserved, relaxing feeling comes when all your muscles, your cells, are feeling fantastic. It's like they've been massaged for an hour! It's as if - no better term I can think of now - all your cells have been replaced, renewed!

In about a year, I got to the point where I was specifically looking forward to the sauna experience! I didn't feel the thirst for fresh air anymore, I didn't suffer and didn't have shortness of breath. There too, I strived for conscious, slow nasal breathing.

I was able to take a sauna while lying down, in fact, I started sweating so slowly, that I voluntarily went up to the higher level bench, because the temperature on the bottom bench was no longer enough! After that, I could hardly wait for the "icy" dive (after a temperature of 80-100 degrees Celsius, the water with +15 degrees Celsius feels icy ☺), and I dived into the water up to my neck without a hiss!

My husband has gone through the same positive changes.

„The real voyage of
discovery consists not in
seeking new landscapes, but
in having new eyes."

(Marcel Proust)

The positive effects
of cold shower

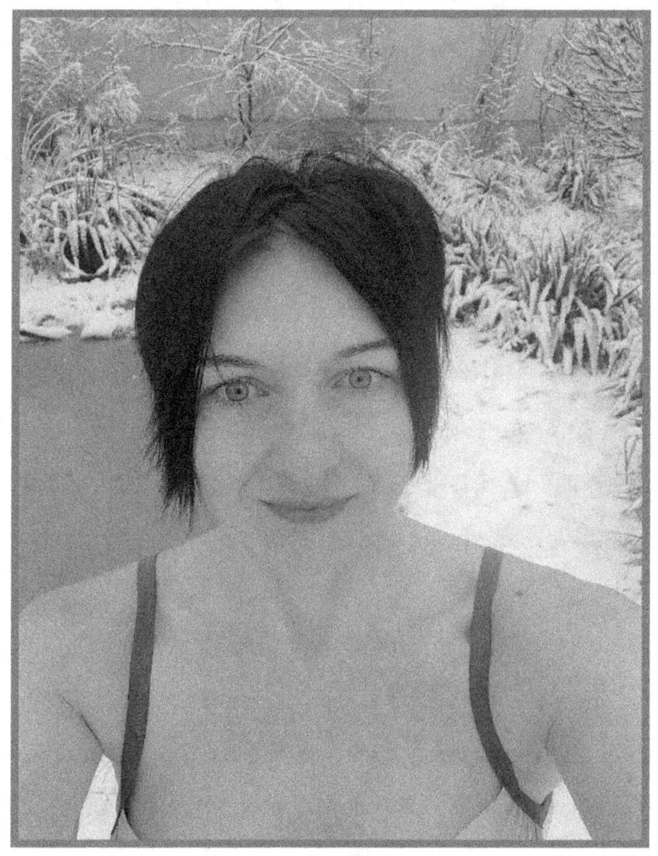

January 25, 0 degrees C, my first bikini walk in the snow!

Let's look at what positive changes the hot-cold alternating shower, cold air therapy and earthing in the winter (barefoot forest walk) brought in my case.

So I started my acquaintance with the cold water with a cold shower. After a "regular" shower I finished with a thirty second cold one. Afterwards, I switched to the three-round alternating shower - started with warm water, always finished with cold water. I did this for a relatively long time, several times a week.

Later, I read that the really tough guys shower with cold water from the start, of course I had to try it right away. ☺

And I did it! I started with cold water immediately, going from ankle to thigh, then two arms from wrist, then abdomen and back, and finally dripping ice-cold water down from my chest! For the sake of "feeling," I also did a hot water alternating shower, and I was terribly proud of myself for being such a hero!

When I got to know Wim Hof's name and discovered Jonna Jinton's YouTube channel, who lives in a small Swedish village of ten and regularly vlogs about icy spring dives, it was time for me to move on: diving into the cold water after a shower! (I definitely recommend watching Jonna Jinton's magical visual and musical videos, this is one of my favorites:

The usual dilemma came of course, how do I get started? Shall I go out into the cold in a swimsuit for a few minutes and settle into a bucket or laver filled with cold water to let my body get used to it? It occurred to me that we have a large plastic bowl into which we fished for goldfish when we cleaned the lake. It's so big that it fits perfectly. Maybe fill it with water and start diving deeper into it every time? I also wondered why should I complicate this, if we don't have a natural lake in the village, here is the pool in the garden! Perfect for practice!

Gradualness is the goal in every case. For some reason I did not immediately think of the most obvious solution: the bathroom tub! For the first time, it is enough to practice diving into cold water at room temperature, then you can vary it in the open air!

So the day came when I half-filled the tub with cold water before the evening shower, calmed my breathing (strictly by nasal breathing), and then started descending into it, pretty slowly, I kept the air in my lungs - otherwise I would not have been able to do it. Slowly but steadily, I didn't stop.

The process of descending was terrible, but after it, when I was fully surrounded by the cold water, the bad feeling turned into a pleasant experience. Practically it feels the same as diving into a pool after a sauna: it doesn't hurt, it's a neutral, relaxing, timeless state!

I didn't know how long it was "necessary" to be in it at first, I didn't want to be ill or possibly catch a cold (even if I know, it's not the cold itself that makes you sick, however your consciousness is able to do it), so I spent 5 minutes in it and stood up. I drained the water and I finished with the usual evening shower. Which was extremely energy efficient as I didn't feel anything on my skin. ☺ Actually it became so insensitive, that I was able to shower in cold water without feeling the temperature. ☺

About the experience itself: I may have already mentioned it earlier, but immersing in cold water alone is much less unpleasant than a cold shower! Contrary to expectations, dipping in half a tub of cold water was a much simpler and more "pleasant" feeling than when I poured cold water on myself. Given the mass of water, it's all up to you: if you decide to dive in without thinking, and then you continue to consciously to stay in, and "tolerate" it.

While in the shower, the cold water zigzags back and forth through your body - I think it also has the advantage, but it is more uncomfortable to live with because it does not cool the skin surface evenly and at the same time, it always "stings somewhere". Depending on which part of your body is being showered. ☺

In summary, experimenting with cold water is absolutely fruitful, it clearly increased my cold tolerance. Diving into the bathtub does not involve any physical and mental shocks, so I am going straight in the direction of diving into the garden pool next winter. ☺

The positive effects of grounding: my first experience was after I returned home from a walk in the cold, that I didn't feel the need to wear socks! Yet I am a cold-handed-cold-legged type. I'm not saying I came home with hot limbs after an hour and a half walk in the forest at zero degrees C! No, everything was ice cold. However, I was more tolerant of the cold every time I walked! It was less and less uncomfortable, more reminiscent of the experience of swimming after a sauna, when I soon got into a calm, quiet, state of relaxation, blinking happily from the cold water like a satisfied hippo at the zoo. ☺

So my cold tolerance also increased clearly and steadily from barefoot walks, and it changed only hours after we returned home: my hands and feet warmed up and poured the heat out of me regularly! So it stayed for the rest of the day, and all night.

It became so permanent (whether it was a barefoot walk that day or not) that I became the official and exclusive bed warmer for my husband, ☺ (of course it was no different before) who was so cold in the bed that he shivered from head to toe under the blanket, while I was already stuffing my limbs out from under the duvet in a pair of panty-jersey, plus I poured heat like a small stove. ☺

Disease - related changes

First of all, I'm basically a healthy person. Twice a year, I tend to "catch a cold" almost on a regular basis, at the turn of the season: once when the weather turns from winter to spring, and the second time from summer to autumn. I have always explained this by the fact that I don't dress properly, I should wear warmer clothes. At such times my throat always hurts for 1-2 weeks, my nose runs, so I chew Strepsils, and I drink Neocitran to cure it.

Furthermore, I also had a febrile illness once a year, always in winter, it passed in 2-3 days, but while having it, I felt: limb pain, weakness, loss of appetite, severe sore throat, and catarrhal cough…

Well, I've haven't had such a complaint for two years! None of them! I eat vitamins, and the duo of a sauna-cold dive, have a role to play in this, plus a year of cold therapy, but overall the strengthening of my conscious thinking. By which I mean that I am increasingly trying to exclude negative thoughts, leaving room for constructive, creative, positive ideas.

I will write more about this in the Chosen Life chapter.

And in general, a few thoughts on the perceptible, positive effects of lifestyle changes - not just in terms of cold therapy. Because since I have been trying to live a healthy life, I have always had doubts – is it worth the investment? So, maybe without losing weight or doing exercises every day, or without applying a gram of moisturizer, I wouldn't have worse lab results or facial skin than now?

It's hard to find an answer to this, because there's no way to live a parallel life and see what one would be like, or check the end result of the other lifestyle…

However, lately I have suddenly received more answers from life. One morning while bedding, I realized that until four years ago, after waking up, I had a regular program to remove my fallen hairs from my pillow!

I also lost a lot while combing as well. I started my second lifestyle change in 2016, and that's when I got used to consuming vitamins and minerals. I did this very irregularly until then. For this reason I also developed abnormal iron deficiency. On the other hand, my hair hasn't been falling for at least 1-2 years, so I have to think, it makes sense to eat vitamins, supplements!

Then I consumed gelatin for a long time to protect and support my skin and joints, and later collagen. Then I had to pause for financial reasons, and I noticed all my body parts were crackling during a workout or when I tried to stand up! For this reason, I also think it is necessary to take both gelatin and collagen!

When I'm "on leave" from a lifestyle change and it is allowed to eating anything, my digestion is completely different than during a balanced diet! At that time, everything inside works "like clockwork" again, so this is a lot of proof that it makes sense to eat well, play sports and live "well"!

And as I wrote in the chapter on grounding, that regular barefoot walking (I think because of it) completely eliminated my morning, post-wake pain in the outer edge of my foot.

"It takes a lot of wisdom
and courage to know which is
the path we want to take and
which is the one we choose
to please others."

(Danielle Steel)

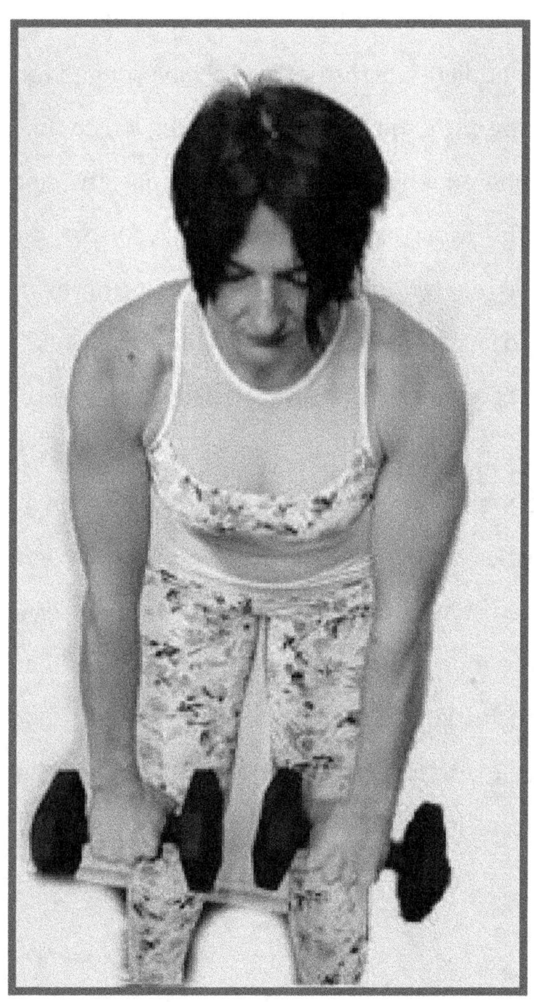

77

As I wrote in my book Fake hunger, I have been training with Anita Herbert since April 2020. She is a Hungarian-born coach currently living in Miami, followed by many-many fans and she has a fantastically composed 6-week training program available for purchase online. By her exercises, I have finally achieved the kind of bodily transformation I always longed for.

I have been training with Anita for a year, during which time I had some interesting experiences. The most important, and at the same time the most exciting discovery was that my muscles "hadn't been created" before. ☺ I'm thinking here, for example, that you do squats as best you can, and then it takes a few months to understand what Anita is talking about — or anyone else who can already do it professionally, what it means to "put the weight on your heels", and how do you squeeze your buttocks when standing up? One fine day you realize that you already have buttocks that you can squeeze. ☺ And if you look in the mirror during your workout, you will no longer see an enthusiastic baby seal, but better posture and the execution of the exercises will be similar to what you see on the monitor from your trainer. ☺ These are fantastic experiences!

And you really don't have to be afraid of weights and dumbbells! Obviously, it's also a matter of genetics, how quickly and easily you get muscled, but at least I think the female body can become beautiful from toned muscles, and that can't happen without lifting weights. I don't mean 100-120 pound weights, I first had 6, 10 and 20 pound hand dumbbells, as well as mini bands and rubber bands, yet I started to take shape. Later, of course, I raised the stakes, squatted with eighty pounds, but even here it is true that less is sometimes more: to load yourself with unnecessary huge weights if you can't do the exercises properly. Rather, it weighs less, but the task is executed perfectly: the result is a wonderful "burning" feeling for the muscles.

I've mastered it and I wouldn't miss the "bottom muscle activation" before training anymore. At first I had a hard time understanding the whole thing, I couldn't implement it (for the reasons outlined above), but as I got stronger, so did the practical enlightenment about what to do. Suddenly I felt exactly the right muscles and I knew also what to do with them. ☺ Activation is necessary in order to really warm up the muscles before the workout, so that during the actual exercises they really need to work.

According to Anita, if you don't feel your muscles while training your buttocks, they most likely won't even work. And then there will be no results.

Finally, what I can definitely suggest about workouts is the use of the SMR cylinder. I use it not only for stretching after workouts, but also for warming up before it. I also do buttocks activation and other traditional "leg" warm-up exercises, but I've found that rolling works with the same efficiency! I feel like after cold water therapies, as if all my muscles have been replaced, refreshed, not to mention that the rate of muscle fever is much lower when I finish my workout with a roller. In fact, I also use it on days off when I'm just so stiff that I can barely walk. ☺

Of course, there are also specifically fun tasks. In Péter Lakatos' book "Timelessly", I read about an experiment - how many of the test subjects (min. 50 years old) can get up from a seat without hands or with the use of one hand? The results showed that those who were able to stand up hands-free or with only a little help were more likely to stay alive the next ten years than those who were not…. Well, of course, at the next family reunion, I had to test it ☺ - even if none of us were fifty - and we all tried the hands-free get-up off the mat.

For my part, I had a lot of fun ☺, one wouldn't even think about how obviously we use our hands and how much we can miss a hand with certain activities!

From then on, I paid special attention to getting up hands-free in all situations: from the chair, sofa, even the bed when I woke up in the morning, from the mat during my workout…. It is very interesting to experience how other muscles engage without hands, but the body adapts quickly. I can only recommend to everyone the practice of hands-free uprising: this is the "workout" that doesn't cost a penny or a separate amount of time, we can practice it continuously in our daily activities. Lessons learned from the experiment, among other things, were that those who were able to get up without support were likely to remain more agile in the following years (bend down for a dropped object or find the slippers under the bed) and thus remain fit and agile.

More information on the topic:

Anita Herbert's Facebook Profile:

https://www.facebook.com/AnitaHerbertFitness

Anita Herbert's website: https://www.anitaherbert.com/

SMR cylinder using video:

Life after dealing with emotional eating

In my previous book "Fake hunger", I wrote about how I identified emotional eating with myself, how I looked for a solution to control it, and then how I applied it. Now some thoughts on what has changed since writing the book, what longer term experiences I have gained yet.

First, the fact voiced by psychologists over time that there is no cure from emotional eating has been fully confirmed, but it can be treated and controlled. This means that if someone, for example, stress, mental upheaval, overload, etc. relieves tension by eating, it may still be the first idea that comes to mind. But it does matter how much "stress-relieving" eating happens and for how long?

I experienced over the months that no matter how long I had been asymptomatic, there were times again when the emotional urge to eat was more pronounced, but I was fortunate to know it and consciously avoided unbridled eating.

I was overeating based on "my own consent," but even then I knew, it would last only for a short period of time.

Another experience is that it is cyclical. It can be 5-6-7 consecutive months without a single emotional eating. Then the "stars change position", things get tangled up and we're more prone to eating too much. But the good thing about this is that we set the rate!

Also, at the very beginning of the treatment methods described in Fake hunger, there is a task where we "learn" to treat food as equals and make no distinction between them in terms of guilt. You can eat sugary food in the same way as salad, the difference between the two is that one doesn't support our weight loss, the other does, but we don't have to feel guilty if we did eat the more harmful food!

However, a few weeks are not enough to fix this! Months later, I noticed that I wasn't really paying attention anymore when I was buying and eating a product based on sugar or flour ingredient: of course, I knew I was not going to lose weight, I wouldn't even keep my weight, I just wanted to be able to eat like I did when I was a child. When I didn't know yet what the weight problem meant. There is only food, delicious, we love it, we eat it, and we don't feel guilty afterwards. ☺

So the most important thing I can say as an adjunct to Fake hunger is that if we are emotional eaters, we will remain so: but that is why if we experience a "relapse", we should not despair, we need to know that this is normal! It's like when someone's "weak point" is their knees: they're used to having nothing to complain about for a long time, but a sudden change in weather or a bad move is enough and limping comes in for a few weeks... You have to learn to live with that.

If we also manage to handle the treatment of emotional eating as such a rippling regularity, I can say that it will be a "smooth affair" to deal with the minor fluctuations that occur cyclically!

Self-knowledge is also a great help. For example, I already know exactly that for me November-December is two months of "let it go". I might be able to change that with great will, but I don't want to. ☺ Because I think that's fine. In preparation for Christmas, it is important for me to taste the flavors and sweets available once a year and eat one of them to my liking! Christmas candy, German honey biscuits, candies, gingerbread... I have noticed that the price of this is that I start with 5-6 kg (11-13 pounds) plus by January, despite all the workouts, but I don't mind.

Because I can already see that I return to my diet without any difficulty every January, and everything continues where I left off at the end of October.

So my lifestyle has evolved from living an exemplary life for ten months, which includes a week of total downtime in the summer when there is no exercise and no dietary meals. But it also fits me to give myself a full two months off half a year later. Training is continuous even then, but there is no explicit restriction on eating. No matter what you employ, the point is to be good for you!

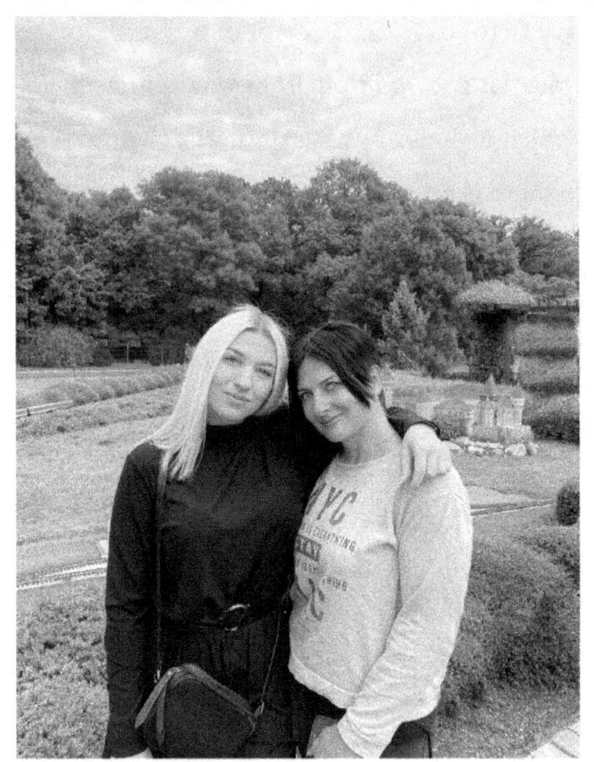

One day you are still young
another day you are
your daughter's sister.

/Patricia Álamo/

www.kilofalo.hu

Facial rejuvenation routine (massage)

I have no objections in principle to cosmetic surgeries, I also had corrective intervention after weight loss because no workout could have helped those areas of the body.

Facial treatment is a bit of a different topic, although I was also interested in it afterwards, and botox was recommended as the most effective for forehead and hyaluron for smile wrinkles. But I don't feel absolutely necessary to have it done yet. Breast deficiency cannot be "filled" in any way like with silicone: there is no form of exercise that can solve the problem. The elongated, flabby skin of a lost belly cannot be "tightened" back with all the collagen in the world, only a scalpel can cut out the excess "residue". But the face? Well, time goes by, there's nothing to do with it, and while you can be pretty sure that the end result will be good for your abdomen, I would be wary of botoxic muscle paralysis because I don't know if it won't get much worse in years to come... Of course, never say never, ☺ but for the time being I have voted in favor of natural, "working" methods.

Years ago, I started looking for massage methods that can be used to keep facial skin young. I selected the most sympathetic, "most livable" method (link to the video later) and started massaging my face on a daily basis.

Face wash

Then, when the alternating shower became a routine in my life, I also got used to cleaning my face every morning with three rounds of hot-cold washes. I also use a face wash soap or facial scrub when I "dip" my face abundantly and thoroughly into the warm and cold water, and every time I close the morning "seance" with cold water. When wiping my face, I rub my facial skin gently but thoroughly with the towel. I do this every morning, approx. for 1 minute, and after I brush my teeth in the evening as well. In both cases (especially since I have specifically dry, sensitive skin), I apply it thoroughly afterwards with a moisturizer.

Lighting

When I met my husband, he brought with him into the common household a Bioptron lamp. I was not interested in the lamp at all, so it moved into a drawer for good. It came to my mind a few months ago because of a shoulder injury and I sat down to find out on the internet what it was good for.

After reading the manufacturer's information about it, I understood that it was good for pretty much everything. ☺ For sports injuries, skin complaints, anti-wrinkle, burn injuries, lightening of surgical scars, sunburn, warts... Well, here I knew that my shoulder was no longer important, ☺ but wrinkles?! This lamp is my "hero"! ☺ I decided to test it as my next experiment in life: it was worth a try! The worst part is that it won't have any effect, but it might even work. So whenever my time allowed, I "lit up". Of course, this is not omnipotent either, there is a lot of information about the Bioptron lamp on the net, if you are interested, you can read about it, they highlight that e.g. it is not a substitute for medical treatment for muscle injuries, but it can be a good adjunct and speed healing.

Face gymnastics

So I did a nice morning-evening, alternating face wash, massaged my face, and used the lamp too, but I thought something was still needed, ☺ and so I found face gymnastics.

https://www.youtube.com/watch?v=Cj9IhMSO9LI&list=PLVB WJW7_KBoHwCTYLuUnYxWNmddzG70WT&index=2&ab_cha nnel=MasumiChannel

https://www.youtube.com/watch?v=RJjHC4JI8R8&list=PLVB WJW7_KBoHwCTYLuUnYxWNmddzG70WT&index=1&ab_cha nnel=MasumiChannel

https://www.youtube.com/watch?v=V4ANcs7oh9s&t=399s& ab_channel=WorkoutVideosX

There is massage in this as well, but also serious facial muscle gymnastics, seriously, in some exercises I almost felt like I was going to have a muscle spasm. ☺

Well, how often do I do these? Face wash in the morning and in the evening. The lighting is approx. every two days and there is a time-saving solution to perform when you are already dealing with your computer or tablet. While lighting, you can read the messages very well (the lamp is in one hand, the mouse is in the other, in fact, I also have a stand for it, so...).

In this case, you can watch development videos, or if you are used to checking a Facebook feed anyway, the 15-20 minutes of lighting a day is a great way to connect the pleasant with the useful.

And I usually do a facial massage in the evening when I watch the actual series on TV with my husband.

After bathing in the evening, I take my jar of moisturizer cream nicely with me to the living room couch, and I have to "massage it through an entire 50-minute part."

The face gym requires a little more organization, namely because sometimes you have to show such a stupid face that it is not possible in front of my other half. That's why I end up either in bed or after waking up in bed (in the dark) or in those (rare) times when my husband has something to do and he is a few meters away from me. ☺

And the most important question is: how effective is it? This is always the hardest one to answer, because we don't know how we would look like without practicing it, do we?

What I do know is, that with my mind today, I wouldn't have grimaced, frowned, "raised eyebrows" as much as I did when I was ten or twenty years old.

(And I think the same about obesity anyway: with my current knowledge, I would have gained up to 30-40 pounds during my pregnancies, not 70. Unfortunately I can't change the past)

What I do know, however, is what comes next! I will most likely not be able to remove (but hopefully I can fade) my already formed wrinkles, which are mainly mimic wrinkles.
But with these home treatments, a lot of hydration, consuming GAL collagen peptide, drinking water, maybe I can prevent the formation of further wrinkles, and that would be a great result!

The Bioptron lamp is the only one of these, which is an extra option from life through my husband, I would never have bought or invested in it myself, but all the others are again just like a hands-free line-up: it doesn't cost money and it's up to us. Whether we invest time and energy to make it a daily routine? About the actual effect of my facial treatment, as well as the meaning of cold therapy, I think we can only get an authentic answer in many years or decades.
Then it will be possible to draw conclusions: will I show more physically and mentally beneficial results than those of my contemporaries who do not train, eat healthily, use cold therapy, grounding, or sauna…. We'll see! ☺

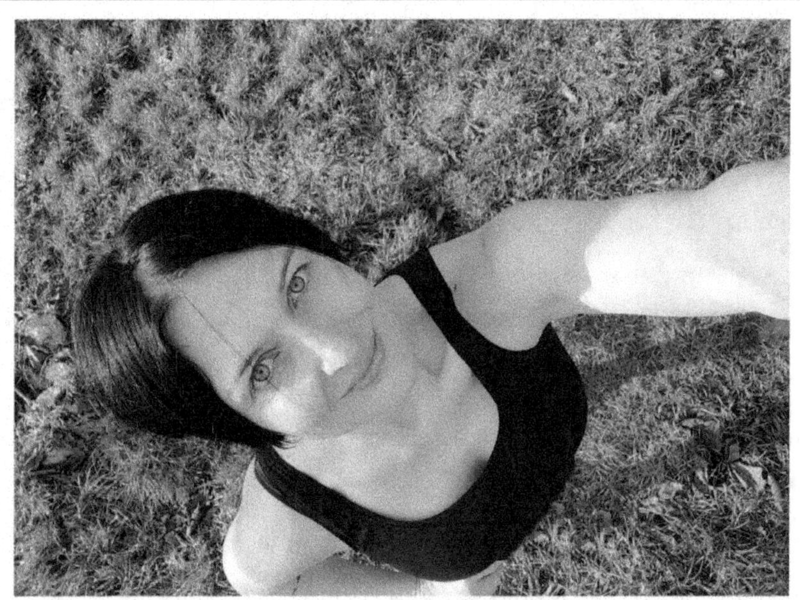

"What you want to ignite in others
must burn in you."
St. Augustine

Covert emotional abuse, narcissistic parent

All my books are about - and this opinion of mine will probably not change anymore - that complete harmony can only be found by the perfect cooperation of body and soul. If my soul feels "good", my body also reflects that. If my body feels "good" (healthy), it shows that everything is fine in my soul as well. In either case, whatever goes wrong, the other "layer" immediately reveals that there is something tangled.

I have several examples and experiences of this in my life. The latest, most recent experience is recognizing and then treating emotional eating. In vain I tried to do everything on a physical level for my weight loss, well-being, appearance that seemed ideal, my soul was not okay and I could not achieve my goal. Unity simply can't exist without both!

In the same way, there was something I realized on the fly, namely, that you can't live a full life, if you are being surrounded by human relationships that constantly spoil or destroy, and don't add to you ...

It is true of this, as well as of emotional eating, that since we have been in it for a long time (even since childhood), we have no idea that this human relationship in question is not normal. That it shouldn't be like that. That not everyone lives like this! That not everyone is treated like that!

I don't want to go too deeply into the subject of narcissism (because that's what it is), but I wholeheartedly recommend György Bánki's thick book, The Greatest Book on Narcissism, to anyone who is interested in the subject.

Almost all of us show narcissistic personality traits on some level, but not to the same extent.

A parent can be narcissistic, or we can experience narcissism in a relationship. What are the key features? Well, there can be quite a few manifestations of this, but the most common is that we live in an *oppressed, sacrificial role toward someone.*

And it can all happen without even being aware that something is wrong around us! For example, if we are born into such a repressive-victim situation! At most, we're amazed that hey, that's what a mom / dad can be like when we get to know our friends 'parents. But we can also experience this through a relationship:

If our parents also lived in a narcissistic relationship, and automatically we continue this line, we may be once shocked that other couples do not behave towards each other the way we have seen and experienced so far...

In general, what makes it suspected that we are victims of covert emotional abuse or verbal abuse? So when the slaps don't fly around us, not even a loud word is heard, yet, is the air around us full of tension, fear, anxiety, and fear of shame?

Such is the case when someone praises and in the meantime he always "stings" there a bit. ☺ And you think you are ungrateful because he certainly didn't mean to hurt you and nothing is good for you and that person deserves a much better child / partner than you! When all the joy you share with him gets a "yes, but" reaction. In the end all your fun and experience of success gets lost and you find it stupid or even embarrassing to mention anything anymore.

Or when you hear "you can't do it anyway", and "it's a good idea, but it won't happen because..." And you also believe that it is really unnecessary to strive for anything, because you are unviable, you can do nothing, you are stupid, worthless...

Otherwise, you are ungrateful, disobedient, others do everything for you, "they live to be good for you," and you are not capable of making such a small sacrifice to give up your dreams for that person, give up having a child, an appointment or a trip...

With such a person, you never know what the next moment may bring! You always watch the mood of the other person (your parent or partner) anxiously, you never have a single quiet moment near you because you never know exactly what mood is he in. What mistake is he going to find in your activities? Are you going to find him in the right mood or in the bad one?

In contrast of course, the other party is free to do anything! He puts you on a pedestal for the slightest trip (e.g., why a crumb is left on the kitchen counter), but if he leaves the table messy out of oblivion, it's a forgivable sin. If you politely talk to a man, you'll be punished by silence for two days while he can flirt with any women.

He makes the rules and changes them flexibly when it comes to himself. You can't make mistakes! You can't go wrong! Never, nothing! You cannot have your own decision, your own will - you depend on him!

You must not do anything, he can do everything and it will never have consequences! There is always an explanation for that.

You may ask, why does anyone tolerate this kind of (sick, distorted) human relationship?! On the one hand, because if it is a child-parent relationship, rebellion does not arise due to the nature of the relationship. Because the typical phrases will prevent you from even trying to do anything against it:
 "- Watch yourself child, who do you think you are talking to?!" or "-Well, don't heat up here for me, while you are living in my house, you do as I say!"
And we'll understand that, he's really the older one, he has the right to rule and that's probably okay anyway. The situation is different in a relationship. There, tolerance can be caused by hopelessness: for example, there is nowhere to go! The reason may be fear: he will find you and everything will only get worse. Maybe you are used to be with that person: well, sometimes he is rude, or gives a slap, he acts or he constantly shames you, but when he is kind, he is so loving! Do you see, how fake this behavior is?

And the reason may be a total violation of self-confidence: I am nobody, I am nothing. If he weren't, I wouldn't be able to live anymore, I wouldn't be able to live alone, I wouldn't be able to find a job, I could stand on my own two feet...

Those who are able to break out of this - because there are people who can - go through a very serious personality development. And step by step, they wake up to self-awareness, stand up for themselves and change. Well, of course, describing this is much easier than actually change. Guilt is constantly working in the victims because narcissistic people are grand masters of making guilt. Even with "small, little half-sentences" stabbed here and there, they can immediately make you feel like an ungrateful bastard, even if you knew half a minute ago that *you* have been humiliated...

If your bully is a parent, it can be a huge barrier to closing a relationship. How would a "good kid," a "decent man or woman," be capable of such horror to turn back on their parent? How to exclude mom or dad from your life? Even if that parent destroys more than he builds and hurts you more than he loves...

"But it's my father / mother!" – you may say. And everything stays the same, but in the meantime, of course, you suffer... On the other hand, the parent we swear allegiance to, despite all their wickedness, can refuse you without thinking - and even more than once... - They can do with us what we are incapable of. They have no doubts like we have about "how could a parent do this to their child?" Well, easily... Luckily, it really does us a "favor" as soon as we get past the first, almost unbearable pain, and we understand it, yes, they threw us away, said no to us. We feel never-never would be able to do this with our own children, we would never be able to hurt, manipulate them - so how is our parent able to do that with us? But then over time, we realize they've done us the greatest favor! The parent made a decision for us that we would never have been able to! It is very difficult for a victim to get rid of their oppressor. In retrospect, however, you may be grateful to be released! All you have to do now is to stay strong and never-ever look back!

Nevertheless, one day you may forgive them, because the feeling of exclusion is bad, and you naively believe that everyone can change! Then after a while, you realize that it starts all over again...

So much so, that the moment may come again when the parent decides we are so unworthy of their love that they no longer want to hear about us! So far, things tend to get worse when something really doesn't happen to the taste of their mouth, when they experience resistance, when we don't dance the way they whistle... The second "denial" perhaps hurts even more than the first one, because here we understand for good: this man / woman doesn't love us! We didn't want to believe this, we didn't want to face it, but knowing how we feel about our children, will make it clear that only someone who feels no love, can repel someone with such a brittle, insensitive heart.

There is one good thing about this realization (in addition to all its pain) that we no longer let the person back into our lives. Of course, you may give an explanation like he or she is sick or had a difficult life. That the parent "didn't mean" to hurt you afterwards. Sure, no one doubts that... But we also have a life that is more valuable than being used as a punching bag or being exposed to the whims of someone.

Finally, another general addition to narcissistic behavior: these types of people always think they are above humanity, society.

They deserve different treatment, royal circumstances, bowing, privileges. They expect extraordinary service, admiration, wherever they appear. Because of them, they can even stop the traffic, interrupt a stage performance, reschedule wedding dates or national events. ☺ Of course, if anyone else were to demand something like this for themselves, it would be outrageous, selfishness, *everything only works in one direction!*

The point of all this is, that if we live in such a relationship and realize it, we can action against it, we don't have to live with it anymore, because this human relationship is destructive and spiritually devours. It prevents you from creating an ideal, harmonious life, just like emotional eating. This needs to be addressed, resolved to get out of it, and from then on we are liberated and "one big step has been taken" towards finding our spiritual peace.

As a closing word, of course the narcissistic line may not only arise in a family relationship. It can be our boss, our neighbor, and even our best friend, our girlfriend...

The main feature of something is not ok, if you never feel good in the company of this person! If there are only "spikes" left in you, or anxiety, shame, overall a bad experience that you chew on for days, then you have no need for that human relationship, so get out of it!

"The only right way is what
works for you!"

(Anita Herbert)

Morning routin

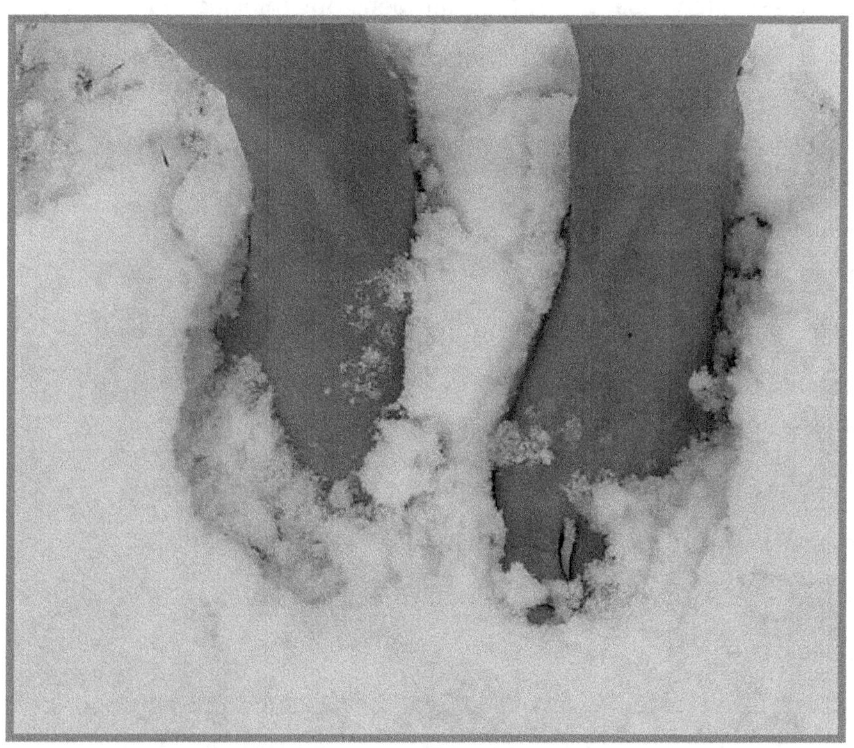

A good morning walk in the snow
right after get up

Visualization (focused meditation)

We have all read and heard that after waking up, we should not immediately reach for the phone-tablet and immerse ourselves in the virtual world that dampens our thinking, but immerse ourselves in our own thoughts, prepare for the day ahead, say positive affirmations about ourselves. Let's give thanks for what we have, let's articulate what else we desire? Let us strengthen our souls, let us be ready to receive all that is good, let us strengthen our bodies.

I don't even bring the phone into the bedroom, except when one of my kids is at a party and I'm on standby if needed. ☺.

In any case, I took the advice, and not only in the morning, but also before falling asleep, in my last sober moments, I always close my day with positive, affirming, planner-creator-grateful thoughts!

I have also created an imaginary world, an island of peace, where my self-guided meditations take place. To give you an idea, I'll tell you what it looks like and how it works.

I'm on a sandy beach. It changes whether it's just dawn or a dark night, and only the light from distant ships is lit on the water surface. There is a beautiful, green, lush tropical garden behind the sandy beach. I can feel the warmth, the sweet scent of the big-flowered, colorful petal plants, the sun on my skin, the touch of the wind. I look up at the sky, wonderfully blue, clear, with snow-white lamb clouds on it. Seagulls howl, the ripples rippling softly, but the water itself is calm, peaceful and crystal clear.

Behind the tropical garden is a castle. It is not large, the castle tower rises in the middle, inside, a staircase leads upwards to the top. I am always there in the tower, from there I look at the wonderful landscape: the garden below me, the sandy beach in front of it, and the endless sea. I rest my hand on the parapet, I feel the roughness of the centuries-old building blocks. I turn around and walk down step by step into the garden. At each round, I pay attention to the ancient stones beneath my feet, which make up the stairs. Old brackets are attached to the walls, the torches inserted in the gloom provide a little dim light.

Arriving at ground level, an arched, large wooden door opens onto the garden, I pause for a moment and sniff a big one from the sweet-salty air. A sidewalk leads in front of me, but it's like a barefoot walkway, the squares of the sidewalk contain different "fillers". As I move forward, I walk on crumbled corn for a few feet, then on small pebbles, then on wood chips, on small twigs - barefoot, of course. ☺

From here, meditation may continue different ways, depending on what keeps my mind occupied. As I stand facing the sea, to my left are rustic, wood-paneled garden shower cubicles, 3-4 side by side.

As I step into the first one, and open the tap, a lukewarm blue beam of light starts flowing on my body, from the top of my head to my ankle. It's a complete cell exchange renewal: as long as it's going on, blue light drips through every millimeter of my skin, every cell in my body is refreshed, rejuvenated and replaced. I move to the other shower, from which green light flows. This eliminates the possible inflammation of my body, my internal organs. I stand underneath and "see" the inflammation appear in red in my body, but where the green light flows through, the red color fades more and more and the inflammation is disappearing.

There is also a "shower" of material well-being and wealth. Of course, liquid golden light is sifting at me. ☺ Delicate lukewarm, running down my face, hair, down every part of my body as I am slowly turning around, coating me everywhere. Then banknotes and gold coins fall on me: I bathe in money. ☺

But I also have an anti-wrinkle ☺ shower with pink light, the possibilities are infinite...

Other times I head to the right where there is a pool of crystal clear water. Whatever I have problem with, the water heals it: I can ask for the ideal look from it, I can to have health, "eternal life". There are times when I look at my current body, my figure, I walk into the lukewarm, beautiful, clear water, I immerse myself, and I come out of it the way I always wanted to look...

You can laugh at this, or you can believe in it. I always look at the benefits. After waking up in the morning, running through political news, horror news, articles that cause anxiety and fear, immediately make me feel bad, or staying in a relaxed state for a quarter of an hour, "dreaming" myself into a warm, friendly, imaginary, reassuring place as a start of the day...

Everyone knows their own answer. ☺

Wake-up air bath

So this - meditation - is my first "morning routine," my second is a three-round alternating water wash, and my third one, in case we don't wake up with my husband at the same time, and I'm the only one moving around in the house, that's when I like to go out to the garden, into the winter cold, wearing only a bikini. In the morning I can withstand the elements much better, it is a massive self-time, the fresh cold is good, the dogs bounce around me, the blood circulation starts, the sun, life… Sometimes I wouldn't even feel like going out in a big jacket, let alone in a swimsuit, but there are days when nothing can stop me from going out. ☺

"Aunt Szoó, what's the secret to a long life?" ☺

I wrote a post in my closed group, and I started it funny: If everything goes according to plan, and I will be 800 years old: one day someone asks me, "Aunt Szoó, what is the secret to a healthy, happy life?" to the best of my knowledge, I would answer something like this:

• "In the winter, you should walk barefoot in the woods at least once a week,

• in the winter, work in the garden for 10+ minutes a day in a jumper and pants

• As many walks during the year as possible

• Breathing through your nose

• Meals within 8 hours a day

• Sauna and swim once a week

• Take a hot and cold shower several times a week

• Train regularly with dumbbells and then stretch

• To do nothing that our body or our soul opposes

• Live so as not to harm ourselves and others

• Eat according to the needs of our OWN body,

• When the time comes, be sure and happily eat a little pastry too! "

And so the post continues:

I've been living by such major points for a long time, they've stacked nicely on top of each other over the years. I got there, even if it contradicts all the logic of the world, and everyone thinks I miss out on the possibility of my life, I still don't take on anything that neither my body nor my soul wants. And I also got to hardest part: to breaking down human relationships that just ruined me. The feeling in my stomach always indicates exactly whether the direction I want to go is good or bad, and I'm just paying attention. Since then, my "freedom" has increased a hundredfold, apart from the minimum necessary to be civilized and live with others, I no longer have to "behave" by raping myself. Assuming, of course, all the consequences and possible difficulties of this, but it was clarified at the basics that "there is no free meal." ☺

And Anita's "Fit in 30" is fantastic! The exercises are so varied, I thought today: for me, Anita's training program is my Advent calendar, 🩶 each day hides a new excitement, I wonder what exercises does it contain? 😄

Chosen life

Over and over again, I have been saying for years now that, my brand "Kilófaló" has meant not just a way of eating, but a way of life that consists of a combination of ideal eating, exercise, physical and mental health. What I stand for, and what I try to "radiate" from myself, ☺ is for everyone to live according to their own desires! Be it eating, sports, human relationships, self-fulfillment, earning money, relationships.

Many, many times - or for a long time – people can't do this, for understandable reasons like e.g. when they have young children and their main task is their care, upbringing, supervision. It's hard to talk about a regular and continuous "self-time" that can stay at the level of desire for years at a time... Or if you want to train five times a week while having health problems, that make even a mere, mundane existence difficult.

These are "lower tiered" states, if the path to happiness is imagined as a pyramid or a triangle. At the bottom, at the widest part, are our most basic needs, at the top, total harmony and happiness.

The rule of life is that until we have completed all the lower level tasks (creating physical and mental health, meeting basic needs (i.e. we are not cold, we are not hungry, we are not deprived, we have a home, we have an income, we are not sick), eliminating addictions, moving up is not possible.

Sometimes we can get stuck in a life situation for years when it doesn't seem like there will ever be a shift. However, if we really want to achieve a better quality of life, it will come true.

I also went through the "I raise my baby-toddler-I travel the country with my books and products — I develop a new product — I write a new book — I cultivate a garden — I keep an animal — I run the household — I try to sort out my first marriage" vicious cycle.

I totally burned out in the process.

I had to admit, despite the greatest desire to give, despite the best of intentions, the day is only 24 hours for me too, and I can't stretch the string any further. At one point I had to say, all together it was too much, and I had to start downsizing.

Since the fundamental problem of my life was the difficulty of letting go, it was very, very difficult to achieve. To end something for good, to say that it is over: to let go of personal or business relationships, activities, to consciously choose to rest, to recognize my withdrawal forces (e.g., the destructive trap of emotional eating).

I had an idea all along about what the ideal life would be for me! This idea has always been with me, even in the greatest of difficulties, because I knew I wanted to get there!

I developed myself, I learned (about myself, about life), I read a lot, I listened to others, I looked for answers, when I found some, I applied them... So the "good life" doesn't fall into anyone's lap, you have to work consistently for it.

However, when you live through the first "upper tier" experience, when it becomes clearer than the sun that you are living a reality that has been visualized for years, only dreamed of it in reality, well, from then on, events will accelerate! ☺ The "vibrations" change, you learn to live in the present, in "NOW", because at once you finally understand what Eckhart Tolle is talking about ☺, you experience the actual creative power of gratitude!

You will learn the three main rules of life that are conditions of happiness:

1. Live in a way that doesn't hurt yourself and doesn't hurt others.

2. If you don't like something, change it! If you can't change it, let it go! If you can't let it go, accept it!

3. Rejoice in what is, do not grieve in what is not!

It is that simple. I deal with issues that affect me personally and I have personal influence over them. What I can't change (destructive phenomena affecting the world, for example) I don't think about them, because they just steal the precious energy, but I can't help those involved in it... According to the very true words of Mother Teresa that "If each of us would only sweep our own doorstep, the whole World would be clean." This means the same, not to rage on things that can't be changed, not to blame others for being there ... but to change what we can... The 3rd thread of my life is that I try to live every single day the way, that if I didn't wake up the next morning for whatever reason, in the evening I would know that everything was perfect in my past day!

I have no sense of lack, I have been with my loved ones (actually or virtually, or in spirit), I have carried out happy, joyful activities, I have solved the difficulties risen, I have learned from them, I have arranged them. This is how you can turn every gray weekday into a wonderful day after a while.

Arriving in the present

I have been looking for happiness for many years. The state where I control my life, I don't have to do anything I don't want, but I can experience everything I desire. I don't have to make destructive bargains, compromises, I don't have to endure the closeness of people who just hurt or take away from me. I can wake up every morning with peace and quiet in my heart, without anxiety or fear of the day ahead of me. I have something - knowledge, ability, experience - from which I can give, which I can share, for the pleasure and support of others. I make sense. My existence has a meaning.

In addition, I am able not to judge people, accept all kinds of otherness and think differently. I am not complaining, I am not rebelling, I do not blame others for making mistakes.

I learn to take responsibility, to be forgiving, patient, insightful and wise…

Who knows when to listen, when to talk (and especially to listen). ☺ He who can handle conflicts, understand the message, and not crucify the bearer of bad news….

To be brave enough to say no while representing my interests if necessary, to learn to let things go, to wait. Have the courage to close human relationships and not remain in destructive situations for fear, or fear of the other's expected aggressive reaction…

And who knows, there is no continuous, eternal "floating" even so! There is cyclicality here as well. From living the infinite freedom and living the life I have been waiting for so long, I know for sure that difficulties will come the same way again, *only to find solutions that are simpler, easier, wiser!*

Achieving these is a lifelong goal. ☺ But I wanted this life, I wanted to become this woman, and even if it seemed infinitely distant, I worked for it every day, to the best of my ability and level of awareness at the time! I searched for the answers and they found me. Once found, I applied them too!

Many, many desperate periods surrounded this path. There were periods of soaring, then came the low point and started all over again…

But I never gave up, even if I wanted to, I wasn't able to, because some inner strength always pushed me forward!

My teacher role models, Tolle, Byron Katie, Mária Szepes, Mother Teresa, Béla Balogh, Ruediger Dhalke, Wayne W. Dyer, Louise L. Hay, were so far away from me. They radiated so much harmony, it seemed at every vibration of their face that they had already transcended the trap of judgment, transfer of responsibility, they were self-identical, and in harmony with themselves and the world! This is what I wanted to achieve, to get here, to polish myself like this, but three, five, ten years ago it seemed so distant, that mortal woman could reach this level.

Then the years went by, a lot of things happened to me, with an awful lot of lessons, insights, "aha" experiences. I had to face my mistakes and bad decisions. I cried myself out, I was ashamed of myself, I regretted them, but soon I stood up and went on with the lesson in mind, making sure I didn't commit these anymore.

Then, after years of hard work, there was once a magical moment when I felt quite accurately and clearly that in that minute the past and the present came together, and I am in a realization that I have visualized as a desire for years! I watered a big flower, it was summer, afternoon, sunshine, loneliness, self-time. Nothing hurt, neither in my body nor in my soul, everything was infinitely peaceful, and just holding a sprinkler tube, standing still, there was an unspeakable euphoria, because it was a perfect moment! Everyone is healthy, we have everything we need, the sun is shining, we have a home, the plants are developing wonderfully - unspeakable! It was the first cathartic experience for me that I was on the right track, my practices and visualizations were working!

It took years until the next similar experience came when I "walked into" a situation that I knew exactly about, "yes it has finally arrived", I'm back in something I've only imagined for years. (For example, you sit in your new car, or hug the Love of your life you've been waiting for until then, or you stand on the beach and your tears flow from happiness to finally seeing the big, blue sea for the first time and being there!)

And the time has come, when after more and more polishing, learning, letting go, insight, forgiveness, and apology, these moments of the past, embodied in the present, have begun to multiply! I have already experienced all of these with my husband, and it has become our habit to say it out loud at such times "my God, this is a materialized moment again!" ☺ We have also thanked for it: we do not call God the force that controls our lives, we simply think without naming it: a guiding Force, a Helping Force, a Supporting Power. Or something like a guardian angel, even if we don't name it, but we definitely believe in a higher level, helping force, and whatever good we experience, we always thank the universe and whatever we would like to have, we ask for support...

We had our first such experience together at the end of summer 2020, and have had been plenty since then! We were convinced about doing something really good in the field of visualization, conscious creation! We both had to let go of our misconceptions about social expectations, learn to take on our real desires! But we were able to support each other, so today we can live the life we've only dreamed of for years, decades!

Anna Zentai a famous Hungarian astrologer wrote about the topic: "In my last post, I compared the experiences associated with this, to a long journey when under the weight of heavy luggage we are crumbling on the road, and we suddenly arrive home to drop the load and feel relief. Even if it was difficult, even if we suffered every single step, we will still experience the moment, when by laying down the burdens, a state of relief, freedom and easy existence will come."

We experience this free and easy existence, moreover together, simultaneously. This especially adds value to the experience if you can do it with the love of your life!

I would add, referring back to an earlier sentence of mine, that this state of easy existence is not a continuous situation in a syrupy, pink mist! But I can really see already, there is no rule that good things in our lives should be automatically followed by bad ones! It is true that life has a cyclical ripple! Up and down, outside and inside, light and dark, cold - warm, with the participation of the opposite poles. But it doesn't really matter whether we stand in the dark with superstitious fear and await the evil that is about to strike after every good period, or whether we are in a state of harmonious existence, ready for more and more evolution.

We know that the experiences and situations yet to come, are opportunities to learn and develop ourselves! It is completely different to consciously wait for the next wave to lift us up, or to stand in fear or just resist with the head stuck in the sand.... Because then, of course, there is no other way to lead life than to force it in the right direction, this is what we call a "blow, a difficulty".

We also have experienced conflict situations, with each other, with ourselves, with others, but now we can deal with them much faster, more effectively, more painlessly, more insightfully and intelligently! Our basic state of existence became the harmony found, but inside always being prepared to receive new lessons. ☺

If for any reason you may think, yeah, well, it's easy for you, because ... Because your kids have already grown up, because you're doing what you want, I'd remind you of the beginning of the chapter. ☺ From the fact that I'm really living the most perfect days of my life now, it hasn't been like this for ten years, five years, but not even two years ... It's good for me now - I got to where I always wanted to be physically, emotionally and well – who can predict that in five or two years you won't be at the same place! ☺

What happened so far is that I have already walked the path where you are still walking: In the beginning I watched in disbelief my role models among my family members, who had already lived their free lives. You know, when your little kid says before going to school: "It's easy for you Mom, you can stay home all day!"

Indeed, but the child needs to be reminded that in his age you went to school the same way, and you lived those years the same way he does now. Then, if he's finished with it, he can stay home or live according to his heart's desire as you do now. ☺

EPILOGUE

Here I'm now. I hope I have been able to pass on everything I have experienced over the last few years. My journey certainly doesn't stop here, I'm moving on, in a beautiful, exciting, new direction! ☺

I recommend my YouTube channel, **Judit Szoó Kilófaló**, where I also tell about my new experiences in my short films. If you sign up, you will definitely not miss anything. ☺

https://www.youtube.com/user/hazisutemeny/videos

Judit Szoó Kilófaló's Official Website on Facebook:
https://www.facebook.com/SzooJuditKilofaloKlub

There is a closed circle where we are like a family, the Kilófaló sympathizers, ☺ readers of my books can get in there, so can you. If you mark me as a friend, I will send the invitation and we look forward to hearing from you.

My official website is www.juditszoo.com
There, you can choose from my books published so far.

If you have any questions or requests, I am always available by e-mail at: hazisutik@gmail.com.

Thank you for staying with me, if you liked it, we'll continue a book later! ☺